MEMBERSHIP REVISION SERIES

100

MCQ's

in

Cardiology

for MRCP Part 1 candidates

Compiled and edited by
JOHN DAVIES FRCP FACC
Consultant Physician
Royal Gwent Hospital, Newport

Davies Publications

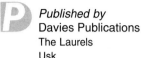 *Published by*
Davies Publications
The Laurels
Usk
Gwent
NP5 1RY

for Astra Pharmaceuticals

This edition published in 1996

ISBN 1 873693 01X

Printed by Chas Hunt,
Cardiff.

CONTRIBUTORS

John Davies FRCP FACC
>   Consultant Physician, Cardiology Department,
>   Royal Gwent Hospital, Newport.

M S Norell MD MRCP
>   Consultant Cardiologist,
>   Hull Royal Infirmary.

C M James MRCP
>   Consultant Physician,
>   Withybush Hospital, Haverfordwest.

A Bokhari MRCP
>   Research Registrar, Cardiology Dept
>   Royal Gwent Hospital, Newport.

Elaine Burfitt MRCP
>   Staff Grade Paediatrician,
>   Royal Gwent Hospital.

INTRODUCTION

The Part 1 of the MRCP examination is a computer-marked multiple choice examination consisting of 60 questions, each with five stem answers which may be true or false. You are allocated a mark for a correct answer and a mark is taken away from your total if you mark incorrectly. If the question is left blank, then a zero mark is allocated.

The exam takes place three times a year at 15 centres in the UK and several centres abroad. Candidates are allowed a total number of four attempts only. There is also a proviso that if a candidate fails very badly, he is not allowed to take the exam for one year.

Candidates are allowed 2½ hours to complete the exam which is usually plenty of time; it is essential that at least 20 minutes be allowed at the end when all the questions have been attempted in order to carefully re-check the answers given.

This is competitive examination with an overall pass rate of approximately 30 per cent. Each exam varies in its degree of difficulty but this is allowed for because more difficult exams have lower pass marks producing a standard proportion of successful candidates for each examination.

It cannot be over emphasised how important it is **not to guess**. Sadly it is well proven that candidates guess incorrectly more often than they do correctly! If you are confident about the answers to 200 stems then it is probably advisable not to go through the exam again adding guess answers. Even allowing a 5 per cent safety margin on the 200 questions this should still leave 180 definitely correct answers which should be more than adequate to pass the examination. On the other hand, if you count your answers and these add up to 170 or below then you have to guess!

Preparation for this examination should include a broad base of reading, including careful perusal of the good quality specialist books advised below. All the big subjects such as Cardiology, Clinical

Pharmacology and Neurology have to be covered but fringe subjects such as Tropical Medicine and Statistics are also included in the examination and when the numbers of these fringe questions are added up, they account for about 30 per cent of the questions.

Attending specially prepared evening or weekend courses where two hours is allocated to each large subject can be valuable, particularly in highlighting areas of poor knowledge requiring further reading before the exam. Such courses can also be very stimulating and certainly less soporific than plodding slowly through a large text book of general medicine.

Actually attempting as many MCQ questions as possible is valuable experience before the examination as this not only gives practice with MCQ technique but also when self-marked can highlight areas of inadequate knowledge. A useful suggestion is to get together into small groups of three or four friends who are all attempting the examination at the same time and to go through a large batch of questions together. This technique is stimulating and time efficient, as large numbers of questions can be covered much more quickly by the 'group brain' than by the individual. Large text books can be on hand to sort out disputed answers.

Standard answers are generally expected for each question and it is probably wise not to become too involved or clever in looking for complicated answers!

In using this book, answers are on the pages directly opposite their questions, to make checking easier. Obviously, this arrangement necessitates covering the right hand page with a piece of card whilst working through the question.

Cardiology is one of the important major subjects covered in the exam and on most occasions there are four or five questions included out of the 60 on this topic making adequate revision mandatory. I hope that the following 100 multiple choice questions in cardiology will increase your knowledge, stimulate further reading and help you to pass the Part 1 MRCP examination.

John Davies

RECOMMENDED READING

TEXTBOOKS OF CARDIOLOGY

The Heart
Hurst J Willis, 6th edition, (1986).
McGraw Hill.

Diseases of the Heart
Julian, Camm, Fox, Hall, Poole-Wilson, (1989).
Bailliere-Tindall, London.

USEFUL SHORT TEXTS IN CARDIOLOGY

Cardiology
Julian D G, 4th edition, (1982).
Bailliere-Tindall, London.

An Outline of Cardiology
Blackwood R A.
Wright P S G.

An Introduction to Electrocardiography
Schamroth L, 2nd edition, (1982).
Blackwell, Oxford.

Essentials of Cardiology
Timmis A, (1988).
Blackwell, Oxford.

Cardiology, (Pocket Consultant)
Swanton R H.
Blackwell, Oxford.

Q1 Coronary artery bypass surgery has been shown to improve prognosis in patients with:

a) significant left main stem disease

b) proximal three vessel disease

c) single vessel disease

d) two vessel disease without involvement of the proximal left anterior descending coronary artery

e) poor left ventricular function (ejection fraction less than 30 per cent)

A1

a) **True**   The Veterans Administration Study in the mid-1970's demonstrated prognostic benefit from surgery in patients with left main stem stenosis of 50 per cent or more.

b) **True**   Prognostic benefit with surgery was also demonstrated in this group of patients in both the European Coronary Artery Surgery Study and the Veterans Study, both undertaken in the mid-1970's.

c) **False**   No study has shown prognostic benefit with surgery in this group. For this reason coronary angioplasty is particularly applicable to this group.

d) **False**   The European Coronary Surgery Study demonstrated an improvement in prognosis, in patients with two vessel disease, if the proximal LAD was involved. For the same reasons as above, coronary angioplasty may be appropriate in this group of patients. However, the role of PTCA in patients with multi-vessel coronary disease has yet to be defined, and may become clearer with the results of randomized studies comparing CABG with PTCA.

e) **False**   Patients with impaired left ventricular function (ejection fraction 35-50 per cent) probably have most to gain from surgery in the presence of three vessel disease, as suggested by the CASS Study. However patients with severely impaired left ventricular function have an increased surgical risk, which counterbalances any potential prognostic benefit.

Q2 Aortic valve closure:

a)   is soft in longstanding hypertension

b)   is accentuated in severe aortic stenosis

c)   is delayed in severe mitral regurgitation

d)   occurs early in severe aortic stenosis

e)   is delayed in left bundle branch block

A2

a) **False**   A2 is accentuated in hypertension as increased systemic vascular impedance produces more forceful aortic valve closure.

b) **False**   A2 is soft or absent in aortic stenosis, although if there is some valve mobility, it may be still audible but delayed. In addition the carotid pulse will be slow rising, and the left ventricular impulse sustained or sometimes double.

c) **False**   A2 occurs early in mitral regurgitation because of shortened left ventricular ejection time. In addition the carotid pulse is of low amplitude although rapid upstroke. This results from rapid left ventricular contraction as a result of ejection into a low pressure system provided by the left atrium. There will be a third heart sound and the left ventricular impulse may be hyperdynamic.

d) **False**   If audible it may be delayed beyond P2. This may cause paradoxical splitting of the second heart sound.

e) **True**   A2 may occur later than P2, particularly in expiration causing paradoxical splitting of the second heart sound.

Q3 Tricuspid regurgitation:

a) has a characteristic appearance on echocardiography

b) is commonly associated with a pulmonary abcess

c) produces a cannon wave in the JVP

d) is associated with ankle oedema

e) commonly produces splinter haemorrhages

Q4 Cor pulmonale is a well recognised complication of the following conditions:

a) asthma

b) schistosomiasis

c) multiple pulmonary oedema

d) oatcell carcinoma of the lung

e) appetite suppressing drugs

A3

a) **False** Echocardiography is not a very precise method of diagnosing tricuspid regurgitation. When combined with Doppler studies tricuspid regurgitation can frequently be demonstrated, but mild regurgitation is commonly found in completely normal subjects.

b) **True** Tricuspid infective endocarditis is the most common acquired form of tricuspid regurgitation. This is especially common in intravenous drug abusers. Septic pulmonary emboli and abscesses commonly occur in this condition.

c) **False** The characteristic wave form seen in the JVP in tricuspid regurgitation is a large V wave and not a cannon wave.

d) **True** Signs of right-sided heart failure including ankle oedema are commonly seen in severe tricuspid regurgitation.

e) **False** Splinter haemorrhages most commonly occur in association with infective endocarditis on the left and not the right side of the heart.

A4

a) **True** Cor pulmonale is a well recognised complication of long standing severe asthma.

b) **True** Involvement of the lung vasculature in schistosomiasis frequently leads to severe and irreversible pulmonary hypertension.

c) **True** Multiple pulmonary emboli may be present with signs of pulmonary hypertension and/or signs of right heart failure.

d) **False** Carcinoma of the lung is never associated with pulmonary hypertension or cor pulmonale.

e) **True** Pulmonary hypertension has been documented to occur as a serious side effect of the appetite suppressing drug Aminorex. It has been suggested that it may be associated with other similar appetite suppressing drugs.

Q5 Typical features of primary pulmonary hypertension include:

a)   chest pain

b)   onset of symptoms in infancy

c)   an ejection systolic murmur at the pulmonary area

d)   a soft pulmonic component of the second heart sound

e)   left ventricular hypertrophy on the ECG

A5

a) **True**   Chest pain, often related to exertion, may be a prominent feature of primary pulmonary hypertension.

b) **False**   The symptoms of primary pulmonary hypertension usually develop during adulthood. A typical patient is a young, acyanotic young woman with shortness of breath, weakness, fatigue and effort-induced syncope.

c) **False**   There is no murmur heard at the pulmonary area. This is a feature of pulmonary stenosis rather than of primary pulmonary hypertension.

d) **False**   Physical signs of primary pulmonary hypertension include:
(i)   a loud pulmonic component of the second heart sound
(ii)   a large jugular venous "A" wave
(iii) a right ventricular impulse
(iv) main pulmonary arterial impulse
(v)   presystolic distension of the right ventricle

e) **False**   The electrocardiograph shows evidence of right atrial and right ventricular hypertrophy. (NB In primary pulmonary hypertension, the strain is on the right side of the heart and not on the left.)

Q6 Ostium secundum atrial septal defect is characterised by:

a) equal sex distribution

b) development of cardiac failure by the third decade

c) a prominent 'A' wave in JVP

d) left bundle branch block on the ECG

e) a single second heart sound

Q7 Antibiotic prophylaxis of endocarditis is recommended:

a) with amoxycillin if penicillin has been prescribed more than once in the previous month

b) after uncomplicated coronary artery bypass surgery

c) in mitral valve prolapse in the absence of a systolic murmur

d) prior to obstetric or gynaecological procedures in patients with a prosthetic valve or previous endocarditis

e) to cover dental extraction or surgery, but not scaling or polishing

A6

a) **False**   The ostium secundum type of ASD is more common in women than in men.

b) **False**   Patients with uncomplicated ostium secundum type ASD usually reach their fourth decade with little or no handicap. Symptomatic infants with early left to right shunts are important exceptions.

c) **False**   The JVP is initially normal with A and V waves of equal height.

d) **False**   Right rather than left bundle branch block is seen with secundum type ASD because the terminal forces point towards the right and anteriorly, producing an "rSr" pattern in Lead V.

e) **False**   Ausculatory signs include a split first heart sound with a loud tricuspid component, a grade II or III pulmonic mid-dyastolic murmur, fixed splitting of the second heart sound and a tricuspid mid-diastolic flow murmur.

A7

a) **False**   In these circumstances Amoxycillin will be insufficient to provide appropriate cover. Therefore Erythromycin is recommended as 1.5g orally one to two hours before the procedure, and 500mg orally six hours afterwards. Alternatively Clindamycin 600mg may be given orally one hour before the procedure.

b) **False**   Coronary artery surgery, if unassociated with valve replacement, does not produce endocardial damage and therefore does not impose a risk for endocarditis.

c) **False**   Mitral valve prolapse is a common clinical finding particularly in young women. It may be apparent as a mid-systolic click and the diagnosis confirmed with echocardiography. However in the absence of a systolic murmur, antibiotic prophylaxis is not recommended.

d) **True**   In patients with a prosthetic valve or in those who have had endocarditis previously, antibiotic prophylaxis should be given prior to obstetric or gynaecological procedures.

e) **False**   Any dental procedure should be covered.

Q8 Pulmonary valve closure:

a)   is accentuated in pulmonary hypertension

b)   occurs early during inspiration

c)   is accentuated in right bundle branch block

d)   is delayed in right bundle branch block

e)   may occur before aortic valve closure in left bundle branch block

Q9 Which of the following statements concerning artificial heart valves are true?

a)   residual gradients occur across artificial valves

b)   embolic problems are more likely to be associated with aortic than with mitral valves

c)   antibiotic cover is required during cystoscopy

d)   anticoagulation is not required with a Starr Edwards valve

e)   haemolytic anaemia has been reported as a complication of normally functioning valves

A8

a) **True** Increased pulmonary impedance results in forcible closure of the pulmonary valve, and thus a loud P2.

b) **False** Increased venous return during inspiration results in delayed pulmonary valve closure. The opposite happens with expiration: right sided flow reduces and more blood is returned to the left side of the heart. Thus left ventricular ejection takes longer and right ventricular ejection is completed earlier, resulting in approximation of the two components.

c) **False** Right bundle branch block results in delayed right ventricular activation and thus delayed P2. However the character of P2 is normal.

d) **True** This results in wide but physiological splitting of the second heart sound.

e) **True** Left bundle branch block results in delayed left ventricular activation and prolonged left ventricular ejection. A2 therefore occurs later with respect to P2, and this results in paradoxical splitting.

A9

a) **True** Small residual gradients are present across most normally functioning prosthetic valves and these can be measured by echo/Doppler.

b) **False** Both aortic and mitral valve replacements can be associated with embolic complications.

c) **True** Antibiotic cover is definitely required for any type of genito-urinary surgery.

d) **False** Following valve replacement with a Starr Edwards valve, lifelong anticoagulation is mandatory.

e) **True** Haemolytic anaemia has been shown to occur as a complication in patients with normally functioning prosthetic valves. It is probably a mechanical complication resulting from red cell damage during normal blood flow across prosthetic valves.

Q10 In patients with hypertrophic cardiomyopathy the following features suggest a poor prognosis:

a)   syncope

b)   left ventricular endiastolic pressure of 20 mm or more

c)   atrial fibrillation

d)   left ventricular hypertrophy with a "strain" pattern on the electrocardiogram

e)   a septal thickness of 20 mm or more in association with systolic anterior motion on the electrocardiogram

Q11 Regarding ventricular septal defects:

a)   small but not trivial defects are associated with an elevated pulmonary vascular resistance

b)   moderately restrictive defects present with congestive cardiac failure in infancy

c)   Eisenmenger's syndrome exists when there is a left-to-right shunt

d)   small defects in the membranous septum undergo spontaneous closure

e)   non-restrictive defects with elevated but variable pulmonary vascular resistance are seldom symptomatic until adulthood

A10

a) **True**   Prospective studies suggest that ventricular tachycardia occurs in subjects who succumb to sudden death and a past history of syncope suggests the presence of ventricular tachycardia.

b) **True**   A high left ventricular endiastolic pressure suggests that the patient has severe hypertrophy and is likely to suffer from heart failure and malignant arrhythmias.

c) **False**   Atrial fibrillation frequently occurs particularly in severe hypertrophic cardiomyopathy, but is not a bad prognostic indicator. Patients often feel unwell when they develop atrial fibrillation, as they are in need of atrial contraction to help augment their usually poor cardiac output.

d) **True**   Ventricular hypertrophy particularly when associated with a strain pattern suggests a severe form of hypertrophic cardiomyopathy with a poor prognosis.

e) **True**   The greater the septal hypertrophy the worse the hypertrophic cardiomyopathy and the poorer the prognosis.

A11

a) **False**   Defects that are small but not trivial at birth are associated with a normal pulmonary vascular resistance, and come to light because of a prominent left parasternal holosystolic murmur that is the only clinical sign indicating a cardiac abnormality.

b) **True**   Patients having moderately restricted VSD with low but variable pulmonary vascular resistance, present with congestive cardiac failure in infancy.

c) **False**   When pulmonary resistance exceeds systemic level, the shunt is reversed, i.e. it becomes right-to-left, and it is this that is known as Eisenmenger's syndrome.

d) **True**   When there is a small ventricular septal defect in the perimembranous or trabecular septum, spontaneous closure is likely, during the course of which the murmur becomes early systolic.

e) **False**   Patients having a non-restrictive VSD with elevated but variable pulmonary valve resistance typically present with CCF in infancy.

Q12 The following features are characteristic of Fallot's tetralogy:

a) a loud pansystolic murmur

b) a loud first heart sound is commonly heard

c) there is a fixed splitting of the heart sound

d) atrial fibrillation is seen in 75 per cent of cases

e) it is associated with increased maternal age

Q13 The circumflex coronary artery:

a) is a branch of the left coronary artery

b) provides branches that supply the anterior interventricular septum

c) provides obtuse marginal branches

d) runs in the atrio-ventricular groove

e) occlusion can cause inferior infarction

*A*12

a) **False**   The systolic murmur heard in Fallot's tetralogy is a pulmonary ejection systolic murmur.

b) **False**   The first heart sound is normal and is either single or closely split.

c) **False**   The pulmonary component of the second heart sound is absent due to pulmonary infundibular stenosis, which is not accompanied by post stenotic dilatation. Fixed splitting of the second heart sound is seen in the ASD.

d) **False**   Atrial fibrillation is uncommon in Fallot's tetralogy.

e) **True**   There is a reported increase in the incidence of this disorder among infants of older mothers.

*A*13

a) **True**   Rarely the circumflex may arise aberrantly from the right coronary artery.

b) **False**   If dominant, the circumflex may give off a posterior ascending branch that will supply the inferior septum.

c) **True**   The circumflex may provide a number of obtuse marginal branches which supply the lateral left ventricular wall.

d) **True**   The main circumflex may run in the atrio-ventricular groove as it gives off lateral branches. This has surgical implications; dissection of the artery in the AV groove is not possible because of its approximation to the coronary sinus, which also runs in the AV groove and may thus be easily damaged.

e) **True**   If the circumflex system provides a posterior descending branch the circumflex is described as dominant. This is found in approximately 15 per cent of the population and occlusion of this vessel will result in inferior infarction.

Q14 The right coronary artery:

a) can be involved in acute aortic dissection

b) provides a posterior descending branch which runs in the atrio-ventricular groove

c) usually provides an atrio-ventricular nodal branch

d) occlusion results in anterior infarction

e) occlusion can result in right ventricular infarction

Q15 The following are helpful in the differential diagnosis of restrictive cardiomyopathy from constrictive pericarditis:

a) a low volume pulse on clinical examination

b) the presence of calcium on the chest X-ray

c) an eosiniophilia

d) echocardiography

e) rapid atrial fibrillation on the electrocardiogram

A14

a) **True**   Inferior infarction can complicate aortic dissection. The left coronary artery may also be involved, but damage of this vessel often results in rapid demise.

b) **False**   The posterior descending branch runs in the inter-ventricular groove.

c) **True**   This occurs when the right coronary artery is dominant as it is in approximately 85 per cent of the population.

d) **False**   This results in inferior infarction.

e) **True**   This may complicate up to one third of interior infarcts and can be responsible for a low output state.

A15

a) **False**   A low volume pulse commonly occurs in both these conditions.

b) **True**   The presence of calcium (which is particularly well seen on a well penetrated lateral film) is virtually diagnostic of calcific constrictive pericarditis.

c) **True**   The commonest cause of restrictive cardiomyopathy in this country is Löeffler's eosinophilic endomyocardial disease and is always associated with a massive eosinophilia.

d) **False**   Echocardiography is notoriously poor in the specific diagnosis of constrictive pericarditis. It may be helpful in restrictive cardiomyopathy but this is not always the case.

e) **False**   Atrial fibrillation may complicate either of these two very different cardiological problems.

Q16 The following may be helpful in the treatment of mild hypertension:

a) salt restriction

b) abstinence from alcohol

c) cessation of cigarette smoking

d) relaxation

e) serum cholesterol reduction

*A*16

a) **True** Salt restriction as a treatment for hypertension is not new. The drastic regime suggested by Kempner in 1948 (rice diet) was very low in sodium. Less severe restriction of sodium intake has recently been reported to lower diastolic blood pressure by up to 10mm Hg.

b) **True** Chronic alcoholism raises blood pressure and abstinence can be effective in restoring blood pressure to normal levels. Excessive alcohol intake can also impair the response to treatment.

c) **False** There is no proof that cigarette cessation will lower blood pressure in hypertensives. However, hypertensive patients who continue to smoke are more difficult to control with drug therapy than those who give up.

d) **True** Relaxation techniques have been shown to lower blood pressure but unfortunately the effect tends to be transitory. Certainly these techniques are worth trying in mild hypertensives and many patients find this approach very enjoyable.

e) **False** There is no proof that lowering serum cholesterol lowers blood pressure. However, in a hypertensive patient, investigation for and reduction of other risk factors for the development of ischaemic heart disease – including raised serum cholesterol – is obviously important.

Q17 Regarding Patent Ductus Arteriosus in a full-term infant:

a) spontaneous closure may occur within one year of birth

b) males are more likely to be affected

c) right to left shunting occurs in 30 per cent of cases

d) there is an association with maternal rubella infection

e) the JVP is elevated even if the duct is small

Q18 Regarding atrial septal defects:

a) the septum primum begins at the endocardial cushion

b) the ostium primum is between the septum primum

c) the septum secundum lies on the right side of the septum primum

d) endocardial cushions give rise to AV valves

e) foramen ovale is the same as ostium secundum

A **17**

a) **False**   In a full term infant, spontaneous closure of ductus is unlikely after three months of age and, in a pre-term infant, closure is unlikely after the first year.

b) **False**   PDA predominates in females with a ratio of 2 or 3:1. Female predisposition is even greater in older patients.

c) **False**   The great majority of patients (95 per cent) with isolated PDA, have left-to-right shunts with pulmonary arterial pressures and resistance considerably lower than systemic levels.

d) **True**   Congential heart disease occurs in approximately two-thirds of offspring of mothers with first trimester rubella infection.

e) **False**   The JVP is normal when the ductus is small.

A **18**

a) **False**   Embryologically, the septum primum begins to grow from the roof of the common atrium.

b) **False**   The ostium primum is between the septum primum and the endocardial cushion.

c) **True**   The septum secundum begins to develop from the roof of the common atrium and the endocardial cushion on the right side of the septum primum.

d) **True**   Endocardial cushions give rise to the anterior mitral leaflet and the septal tricuspid leaflet.

e) **True**   Ostium secundum is also known as the foramen ovale.

Q19 The left anterior descending coronary artery:

a) supplies the posterior left ventricular wall

b) occlusion results in anterior infarction

c) supplies the majority of inter-ventricular septum

d) supplies the left ventricular apex

e) runs in the posterior inter-ventricular groove

*A*19

a) **False** This is supplied by either the right or circumflex arteries, depending on dominance, which provides the posterior descending branch.

b) **True** The size of anterior infarction with LAD occlusion depends largely on the size of the LAD and the site of occlusion. Proximal LAD occlusion produces a large antero-lateral infarct because septal branches and diagonal branches are also compromised. This may carry a high mortality. Alternatively occlusion of the LAD distal to septal and diagonal branches may result in a relatively localised apical infarct.

c) **True** Septal branches perforate the septum and supply the anterior two thirds. Disease in the septal branches themselves is not amenable to bypass grafting although rarely angioplasty may be tried here.

d) **True** Distal LAD occlusion may result in apical infarction. Because basal contraction is well preserved there may be increased tendency to left ventricular aneurysm formation in this circumstance.

e) **False** The posterior descending branch of either the right or a dominant circumflex system will run in the posterior inter-ventricular groove. However the LAD runs in the anterior inter-ventricular groove.

Q20 Regarding cardiac investigation and intervention:

a) cardiac catheterization in most centres carries a mortality of 5 per cent

b) aortic valve replacement in an otherwise fit patient carries a mortality of 20 per cent

c) coronary angioplasty is usually performed under general anaesthetic

d) coronary angioplasty is contraindicated in multi-vessel disease

e) the saphenous vein has a better long term patency rate than the internal mammary artery graft.

*A*20

a) **False**   Most centres would have a mortality rate of between 1 in 1,000 and 1 in 2,000.

b) **False**   The mortality for aortic valve replacement should be less than 5 per cent.

c) **False**   Angiography and angioplasty are local anaesthetic procedures. This is because the patient can then tell the operator whether or not he is experiencing chest discomfort. Secondly the patient may be required to perform manoeuvres, e.g. deep inspiration which will assist fluoroscopy. Thirdly general anaesthetics, which themselves carry a risk, may produce haemodynamic abnormalities which may not be desirable in patients with cardiac disease.

d) **False**   A third to half of all angioplasty procedures are performed on patients with multi-vessel disease. The place of angioplasty in single vessel disease is clear although its role in multi-vessel disease has yet to be defined. This will become clearer when the results of studies comparing coronary artery surgery with PTCA in these patients, are available.

e) **False**   Ninety per cent of internal mammary artery grafts are patent at 10 years. In comparison 15 per cent of vein grafts are occluded after the first year, and there is an attrition rate of approximately 2 per cent per year.

Q21 Regarding coronary artery bypass surgery:

a) only patients who have received thrombolytic therapy should be considered for early surgery

b) surgery improves left ventricular function

c) prognosis is improved in asymptomatic patients with 3 vessel disease

d) surgery improves prognosis in patients with left main stem disease

e) this procedure cannot be performed in patients who have severe varicose veins

Q22 Regular amiodarone therapy may be associated with the following complications:

a) skin discoloration

b) lung fibrosis in 5 per cent of patients treated

c) abnormalities of thyroid function tests without thyroid disease

d) prolongation of the QT interval

e) reduction of the serum digoxin level

*A*21

a) **False**   Surgery should only be considered following thrombolisis in patients who have continuing severe angina resistant to medical therapy, or when they have positive changes early on during exercise testing.

b) **False**   There is no proof that coronary artery bypass surgery improves left ventricular function; it may, however, stop it getting worse.

c) **False**   The answer to this question is unknown, as all current studies comparing the results of medical and surgical treatment are based on patients with angina.

d) **True**   It has been established that patients with left main stem disease live longer if they are treated surgically rather than medically.

e) **False**   Although leg veins are normally used for the bypass procedure, the presence of varicose veins does not exclude the patient from surgery. Internal mammary artery grafts are frequently used and arm veins may be harvested instead of leg veins. Plastic shunts have also been used instead of veins in this technique.

*A*22

a) **True**   Slatey grey skin discoloration is common in patients on long term amiodarone. This drug is also associated with photosensitivity.

b) **False**   Lung fibrosis is a rare complication of long term, very high dose amiodarone therapy.

c) **True**   Amiodarone displaces thyroxine from serum albumin and will frequently result in high serum levels of T4 when the ''Free T4'' may be completely normal. On the other hand amiodarone is associated with actual thyrotoxicosis and may also produce myodema particularly in elderly patients with high TSH levels.

d) **True**   Amiodarone therapy is associated with prolongation of the QT interval.

e) **False**   Again by displacement, amiodarone increases rather than decreases the free digoxin level. When this therapy is initiated, most physicians advise a 50 per cent reduction in digoxin intake if the patient is already on this therapy.

Q23 Features of coarctation of the aorta include:

a) hypertensive retinopathy commonly revealed by fundoscopy

b) males are more affected

c) there is an association with Down's syndrome

d) a prolonged PR interval

e) absent femoral pulses

Q24 The following features at birth may indicate a diagnosis of congenital heart disease in a full term infant:

a) neonatal cyanosis

b) congenital asplenia

c) polysplenia

d) transverse liver

e) situs inversus

*A*23

a) **False**   Fundi rarely show hypertensive retinopathy but occasionally display U-shaped or corkscrew retinal arteries.

b) **True**   This condition predominates in males with a sex ratio as high as 3:1.

c) **False**   Turner syndrome rather than Down's syndrome is associated with coarctation.

d) **False**   The PR interval is always within normal limits.

e) **True**   The hallmark of coarctation is systemic hypertension and abnormal differences in upper and lower extremity pulses. Femoral pulses are either absent or reduced.

*A*24

a) **True**   Neonatal cyanosis develops whenever there is a right to left shunting of the blood, e.g. Fallot's tetralogy.

b) **True**   Congenital asplenia is associated with various cardiac anomalies, such as dextrocardia, levocardia and TAPV connection.

c) **True**   Congenital polysplenia, like asplenia, is associated with cardiac anomalies such as partial APV connection and absent coronary sinus.

d) **True**   Transverse liver may be a feature of cardiac malposition such as meso or dextrocardia.

e) **True**   Situs inversus usually accompanies dextrocardia.

Q25 In valve surgery:

a) a xenograft makes mechanical opening and closing sounds

b) the Bjork-Shiley valve is a widely available ball and cage prosthesis

c) a homograft is a sterilized porcine valve

d) anticoagulation is not required after mechanical valve replacement if the patient is in sinus rhythm

e) following valve replacement with a prosthesis, there is little further risk of endocarditis

*A*25

a) **False**   A xenograft is a tissue valve derived from an animal source. The most commonly available xenografts are porcine valves mounted on a wire stent, e.g. the Carpentier-Edwards valve. These produce heart sounds that are indistinguishable from normal. They tend not to last as long as mechanical valves, but have the advantage of not requiring anticoagulation with Warfarin. Warfarin may be required for the first three months after insertion to allow for valve endothelialisation.

b) **False**   This is a tilting disc valve which tends to produce only a prosthetic closure sound. The use of this type of valve rather than a Starr-Edwards valve is usually at the discretion of the surgeon. However both require anticoagulation with warfarin.

c) **False**   This is derived from a human cadaver, rather than a pig source. Aortic homografts are not commonly used at present because they require more surgical skill to insert. Some series suggest that they tend not to last as long as mechanical valves, but have the advantage of not requiring anticoagulation.

d) **False**   The insertion of any mechanical valve requires lifelong anticoagulation. This is one important factor in determining the type of valve to be inserted. A young patient would be suitable for a mechanical valve as it may be preferable to avoid a second operation if possible. However women who are planning pregnancy may be given a tissue valve, so as to avoid treatment with warfarin. This may then be electively replaced when her family is complete. Each case requires individual assessment and discussion with the surgeon.

e) **False**   The presence of a prosthetic valve does not remove the risk of endocarditis. Furthermore endocarditis on a prosthetic valve is a particularly serious condition with a high mortality.

Q26 Following uncomplicated aortic valve replacement with a Starr-Edward's valve, auscultation would normally reveal:

a) a prosthetic first sound

b) an aortic opening sound

c) an ejection systolic murmur

d) a prosthetic second sound

e) an early diastolic murmur

Q27 Which of the following are contra-indicators to beta blocker therapy:

a) Raynaud's phenomena

b) Parkinson's disease

c) asthma

d) intermittent claudication

e) Wolff-Parkinson-White syndrome

*A*26

a) **False**   The first sound is physiological representing mitral and tricuspid valve closure.

b) **True**   This prosthetic sound is often mistaken for the first heart sound which occurs earlier. It results from the ball being thrown against the top of the cage during left ventricular ejection.

c) **True**   It is common to pick up systolic murmurs due to turbulence through the cage and round the ball.

d) **True**   As left ventricular pressure falls the ball falls back into the sewing ring, closing the valve and producing a prosthetic second sound.

e) **False**   This would indicate aortic regurgitation through a para-valvar leak. This should be a concerning finding and suggests dehiscence of the valve ring or endocarditis.

*A*27

a) **True**   A vasospastic condition such as Raynaud's phenomena frequently gets worse on beta blocker therapy.

b) **False**   There is no evidence that this therapy influences the development or the progression of Parkinson's disease.

c) **True**   Asthma and chronic obstructive airways disease are specific contraindications to beta blocker therapy.

d) **True**   Patients with angina and intermittent claudication frequently complain that their claudication gets worse when they start beta blocker therapy. When angina patients have this complication, nitrates and/or calcium antagnonist drugs are preferable.

e) **False**   Beta blockers are not contraindicated in Wolff-Parkinson-White syndrome. The only drug to be specifically avoided is digoxin.

Q28 Which of the following features support the diagnosis of acute rheumatic fever:

a) Huntington's Chorea

b) erythema induratum

c) haematuria

d) polyarteritis

e) Osler's nodes

Q29 The following are congenital acyanotic cardiac diseases without a shunt:

a) ostium primum defect

b) coronary arteriovenous fistula

c) pulmonary stenosis with VSD

d) pulmonary AV fistula

e) aortopulmonary window

*A***28**

a) **False** Huntington's Chorea is a dominantly inherited condition which occurs in males and produces presenile dementia – it is nothing to do with rheumatic fever.

b) **False** Erythema marginartum and not erythema induratum is the rash frequently seen in children with rheumatic fever.

c) **False** The kidneys are not involved in the acute rheumatic process and haematuria is not a feature of this disease.

d) **True** Polyarteritis is the usual presenting symptom in adults with rheumatic fever. This is often migratory affecting the large joints especially the knees, elbows, ankles and wrists.

e) **False** Osler's nodes are small painful raised red lumps that usually occur on the pulp of the fingers in infective endo-carditis. These lesions are probably immunologically mediated although bacteria have been isolated from them. They are not seen in rheumatic fever.

*A***29**

a) **True** In ostium primum ASD there is left to right shunting, therefore there is no cyanosis.

b) **True** There is a shunt between the aortic root and right side of the heart, which includes coronary AV fistula; this is characteristically acyanotic.

c) **False** Pulmonic stenosis with VSD (Fallot's tetralogy) leads to a right-to-left shunting because of obstruction to right ventricular outflow.

d) **False** In the case of pulmonary AV fistula there is a normal left ventricle and right ventricle, but a communication at the pulmonary vasculature level leads to cyanosis.

e) **True** There is a shunt between the aorta and pulmonary trunk. The flow is still left-to-right, therefore no cyanosis occurs.

Q30 The following are suggestive of congenital complete heart block:

a) maternal SLE

b) maternal antibodies to ribonucleo protein Anti Ro (SS-A)

c) a family history of complete heart block

d) a normal exercise tolerance in the affected individual

e) a maternal history of Stoke Adams attacks

Q31 Recognised postoperative complications of coronary artery bypass grafting include:

a) stroke

b) endocarditis

c) atrial fibrillation

d) heart block

e) pericardial effusion

A30

a) **True** Maternal connective tissue diseases, especially but not exclusively SLE, are of recognised etiological importance in the pathogenesis of congenital complete heart block.

b) **True** Maternal auto antibodies to ribonucleo protein Anti Ro (SSA) are serological markers of the risk of congenital heart block.

c) **True** Familial complete heart block is well recognised and has been detected in parents of affected siblings. There is also risk of female predominance.

d) **True** The patients have a normal or nearly normal exercise tolerance. One patient was an ardent hockey player and others have included an air force pilot and a cricket player.

e) **False** Stoke Adams attacks are seen in the affected child and not in the mother.

A31

a) **True** This is a particular risk in patients with known cerebrovascular disease.

b) **False** Coronary artery surgery does not impose a risk of endocarditis as the endocardium is not affected.

c) **True** This often occurs after cardiac surgery and may be related to pericardial irritation.

d) **True** This may occur as a result of prolonged cardioplegia or perioperative infarction.

e) **True** This may rarely require drainage because of tamponade.

Q32 Epidemiology of coronary artery disease:

a) the mortality risk from coronary artery disease increases with increasing diastolic blood pressure, but not with increasing systolic blood pressure

b) there is a higher mortality for coronary artery disease in social class 1 than in social class 5

c) discontinuing cigarette smoking reduces the risk of coronary artery disease mortality

d) the risk of coronary disease mortality is proportional to the level of serum high density lipoprotein

e) blood pressue reduction has been shown to reduce the risk of mortality from coronary artery disease

Q33 Doppler echocardiography can be used to:

a) differentiate innocent from pathological murmurs

b) evaluate prosthetic valve function

c) estimate cardiac output

d) estimate intra-cardiac pressures

e) detect and quantify stenotic valvular lesions

*A***32**

a) **False**   The risk of coronary disease increases with both systolic and diastolic blood pressure.

b) **False**   The risk is higher in social class 5.

c) **True**   The risk of coronary disease decreases over a few years after discontinuing smoking.

d) **False**   The risk is inversely proportional to the level of HDL. However as HDL accounts for only a minority of the total cholesterol this does tend to reduce the significance of an elevated level of total cholesterol.

e) **False**   Blood pressure reduction has been shown to reduce the instance of stroke, but not of myocardial infarction. There may be a number of reasons for this. It has been suggested that the beta blocker drugs used in some of the studies may have adversely affected lipid profiles, thus potentially increasing the risk of coronary disease.

*A***33**

a) **True**   This technique can be particularly useful in reassuring pregnant women with benign physiological flow murmurs.

b) **True**   The most useful technique in this situation is transoesophageal echocardiography, but standard investigations are also useful in determining prosthetic valve function and excluding thrombus formation.

c) **True**   This technique is as good in determining cardiac output as any other, i.e. ventriculography, contrast ventriculography and isotope measurements.

d) **True**   End diastolic pressures can be measured and pulmonary artery pressure can also be calculated by Doppler echocardiography, which may be a particularly useful evaluation in assessing the severity of valvular lesions.

e) **True**   The presence of mitral and aortic valve stenosis can be ascertained by echocardiography, and the severity of the gradient across the stenosed valves can be measured non-invasively by Doppler.

Q34 During exercise testing:

a) U wave inversion is not usually significant

b) hyperventilation may induce ST segment depression

c) a fall in systolic BP on exercising is not usually significant

d) ST depression is the most useful sign of myocardial ischaemia

e) ischaemic changes may occur after the patient has stopped exercising

Q35 In infective endocarditis:

a) echocardiography is the best diagnostic aid

b) alpha-haemolytic streptococci are the most common causative organisms

c) prophylactic tetracycline is indicated prior to dental treatment

d) acute surgery of a severely affected valve may be a life saving procedure

e) it is sometimes seen to occur on a completely normal heart valve

*A*34

a) **False**   U Wave inversion has been suggested to be an insensitive but quite specific marker for left anterior descending artery stenosis.

b) **True**   Hyperventilation may induce ST segment depression, probably through a reduction in vagal tone.

c) **False**   A fall in systolic blood pressure by 10 mm of mercury, or failure to rise above 130 mm of mercury may be an early marker of significant ischaemic heart disease produced by left ventricular dysfunction, which becomes more marked on exercise.

d) **True**   Although ST segment depression is the most useful sign of myocardial ischaemia, ST segment elevation can occasionally occur and the development of left bundle-branch block or multiple extrasystoles are also thought to be diagnostic of ischaemic heart disease.

e) **True**   It is very important to monitor the electrocardiogram carefully in the recovery period as ischaemic ST segment changes may occur in this period which have not been manifest during exercise.

*A*35

a) **False**   A normal echocardiogram does not exclude infective endocarditis. Blood cultures are by far the most important investigation in this condition. Vegetations if present can be a helpful diagnostic and prognostic indicator.

b) **True**   Streptococci are still the commonest organisms cultured.

c) **False**   Bacteriocidal antibiotics should be used rather than tetracycline which is bacteriostatic. The recommended therapy is a 3g sachet of amoxicillin in adults unless they are allergic to penicillin, when erythromycin should be used.

d) **True**   Valve replacement should be considered at any stage in the treatment of infective endocarditis and may be a life saving procedure in patients with severe valve destruction causing acute heart failure.

e) **True**   Infective endocarditis has been well documented to occur on completely normal heart valves.

Q36 Aortic stenosis:

a) causes fixed splitting of the second heart sound

b) often produces a thrill in the supra sternal notch

c) is likely to be severe if there is considerable left ventricular hypertrophy with a ''strain'' pattern on the electrocardiogram

d) is unlikely to be severe if the blood pressure is normal

e) is most commonly associated with a previous history of rheumatic fever in UK patients

A36

a) **False** Fixed splitting is never heard in aortic stenosis. This is most commonly found in atrial septal defects. Aortic stenosis most commonly produces reverse splitting or a single second heart sound.

b) **True** Aortic stenosis is often associated with a thrill which is frequently better palpated over the suprasternal notch rather than over the aortic area of the anterior chest wall.

c) **True** A left ventricular strain pattern seen on the electrocardiogram is an indication that the aortic valve gradient is high and that the aortic valve stenosis is severe.

d) **False** Blood pressure is an unreliable guide to the severity of aortic stenosis especially in elderly patients. Pulse characteristics are a much better guide; aortic stenosis is frequently associated with a slow rising pulse. Severe aortic stenosis can occur in combination with hypertension.

e) **False** In the United Kingdom congenital bicuspid calcific aortic stenosis is by far the commonest cause of this condition.

Q37 In the normal cardiac cycle:

a) mitral valve opening occurs simultaneously with aortic valve closure

b) left ventricular filling is largely complete before atrial systole

c) the aortic valve opens simultaneously with mitral valve closure

d) the aortic valve opens at peak left ventricular pressure

e) the dicrotic notch on the arterial pressure wave form is simultaneous with aortic valve closure

Q38 The jugular venous pulse:

a) inspection of the normal adult normally reveals A, C and V waves

b) the X descent results from downward displacement of the AV valves during ventricular systole

c) the V wave results from atrial filling during ventricular systole

d) the Y descent begins with opening of the AV valves

e) the physiological third sound may be heard synchronous with the X descent

A37

a) **False**   Mitral valve opening is delayed after aortic valve closure, as left ventricular pressure falls during isovolumic relaxation.

b) **True**   Atrial contraction contributes approximately 15 per cent to end diastolic left ventricular filling. However the loss of atrial systole may have serious consequences for patients in whom the filling is impaired due to decreased left ventricular compliance, e.g. hypertrophic cardiomyopathy.

c) **False**   Aortic valve opening is delayed after mitral closure, as left ventricular pressure rises during isovolumic contraction.

d) **False**   The aortic valve opens when left ventricular pressure exceeds aortic diastolic pressure.

e) **True**   Aortic valve closure produces a rebound pressure wave apparent as a dicrotic notch. In young individuals or those with hyperdynamic circulations, this may be palpable at the wrist.

A38

a) **False**   The C wave is not normally appreciated. This occurs as a result of tricuspid valve closure which causes a slight elevation in right atrial pressure. The A wave is the result of atrial systole, and the V wave the result of increasing atrial pressure as the right atrium fills against a closed tricuspid valve.

b) **True**   Ventricular systole produces slight enlargement of right atrial dimensions and thus a transient fall in right atrial pressure.

c) **True**   During ventricular systole, the atrium is filling against a closed AV valve.

d) **True**   As the tricuspid valve opens the right atrium empties and pressure falls. This may be particularly rapid in cases of pericardial constriction.

e) **False**   The third heart sound is produced by rapid filling in early diastole, i.e. associated with the Y descent.

*Q*39 Mitral valve prolapse:

a)   when visible on echocardiography is likely to produce symptoms

b)   can occasionally cause an early diastolic murmur heard at the apex

c)   is often introduced by a click

d)   can be complicated by infective endocarditis

e)   is found on echocardiography in 12 per cent of the normal population

*Q*40 The murmur of mitral valve prolapse becomes louder during:

a)   amyl nitrate inhalation

b)   the straining of the valsalva manoeuvre

c)   standing from the supine position

d)   acute anxiety

e)   an infusion of salbutamol

A39

a) **False**   Mitral valve prolapse is not commonly associated with any clinical symptoms.

b) **False**   The murmur heard in mitral valve prolapse is a late systolic murmur and this valve lesion does not produce any early or late diastolic murmurs.

c) **True**   The most common auscultatory finding in mitral valve prolapse is that of a mid systolic click followed by a late crescendo systolic murmur.

d) **True**   There have been many documented cases of infective endocarditis complicating mitral valve prolapse. Therefore in this condition dental antibiotic prophylaxis is essential.

e) **False**   Approximately 4 per cent of the population have mitral valve prolapse.

A40

a) **False**   The murmur of mitral valve prolapse becomes softer rather than louder during amyl nitrate inhalation and the straining of the valsalva manouevre. This is a result of the decreased left ventricular end diastolic volume and associated hypotension during both of these procedures.

b) **False**   See *a)* above.

c) **True**   On standing the murmur becomes longer and louder.

d) **True**   During acute anxiety, the murmur occurs earlier and becomes longer and louder.

e) **True**   Infusions of sympathomimetic drugs have the same effect on the murmur of mitral valve prolapse as acute anxiety.

Q41 Regarding digoxin:

a)   digoxin dosage should be influenced by renal function

b)   digitoxin has a shorter half life elimination than digoxin

c)   digoxin toxicity can be precipitated by hypokalaemia

d)   it is unnecessary to stop digoxin prior to DC conversion of fast atrial fibrillation

e)   digoxin overdose is the commonest cause of supraventricular tachycardia with AV block

Q42 The following are diagnostic of carditis in acute rheumatic fever:

a)   choreaform movements

b)   a mid diastolic murmur heard best in the mitral area

c)   a tachycardia associated with an aortic ejection systolic murmur

d)   prolongation of the PR interval on the electrocardiogram

e)   an aortic early diastolic murmur

*A*41

a) **True**   Renal excretion is the main elimination route of digoxin and therefore dosages should be reduced in the presence of impaired kidney function.

b) **False**   Digitoxin has a half life of approximately 6 days while that of digoxin is nearer 2 days in the presence of normal kidney function.

c) **True**   Digoxin toxicity is much more common in the presence of a low serum potassium.

d) **False**   It is usual to stop digoxin for 24 hours before cardioversion as digoxin toxicity has been associated with ventricular fibrillation precipitated by DC shock

e) **True**   In the elderly digoxin toxicity particularly in the presence of impaired kidney function or a low potassium is the commonest cause of this arrhythmia.

*A*42

a) **False**   Choreaform movements certainly occur in rheumatic fever but they are not definite evidence of cardiac involvement.

b) **True**   The so called "Carey-Coombs" mid diastolic mitral murmur is diagnostic of mitral valvulitis.

c) **False**   Tachycardia associated with an aortic ejection flow murmur can occur in any pyrexial illness and is certainly not diagnostic of acute rheumatic fever.

d) **True**   A prolonged PR interval is a recognised "minor" criteria for the presence of cardiac involvement in rheumatic fever.

e) **True**   The presence of acute aortic incompetence is diagnostic of cardiac involvement in acute rheumatic fever.

Q43 During cardiac arrest, electro-mechanical disassociation may be due to:

a) pericardial tamponade

b) pneumothorax

c) hypokalaemia

d) acute massive pulmonary embolism

e) digoxin toxicity

A43

a) **True**   This may be suspected by an elevated venous pressure and pulsus paradoxus. The preceding ECG may reveal low voltage complexes (less than 5 mm deflection in the standard leads), and the diagnosis is confirmed with echocardiography. Emergency pericardial aspiration may be required.

b) **True**   Tension pneumothorax may distort the mediastinum leading to impaired cardiac function. This should be considered after transpleural or bronchoscopic procedures and confirmed on X-ray. Tracheal deviation away from the affected lung and a hyper-resonant percussion note should suggest the diagnosis. Insertion of a small calibre cannula may be lifesaving in these circumstances.

c) **False**   Although hypokalaemia may distort the QRS complex it does not affect ventricular mechanics. This is therefore not a cause of electromechanical disassociation.

d) **True**   This should be considered in susceptible patients, i.e. post operative cases. It may be suggested by collapse associated with an elevated venous pressure, shock and a right ventricular gallop rhythm. The ECG may show new right axis deviation and right bundle branch block configuration and sometimes atrial fibrillation. Cardiac massage in these cases may break up the pulmonary clot and restore circulation, but emergency pulmonary embolectomy is the only definitive therapy.

e) **False**   Digoxin toxicity may produce arrythmia but ventricular contraction is not specifically impaired.

Q44 Cigarette smoking:

a) is more common in social class 5, compared to social class 1

b) accounts for one quarter of coronary fatalities in men and women under 65

c) increases the overall risk of death to twice that of non-smokers

d) is commoner in Scotland than in the south west of England

e) is increasing in the general population

A44

a) **True**   This may be a reason why the mortality rate for coronary disease in social class 5 is not falling as fast as in social class 1.

b) **True**   Smoking increases the risk of myocardial infarction. In men, 25 per cent of coronary deaths, and in women 20 per cent can be attributed to smoking.

c) **True**   Ischaemic heart disease is five times more common in male smokers compared to non-smokers. Carcinoma of the bronchus is almost exclusively a disease of smokers.

d) **True**   In Scotland, 35 per cent of the population smoke, compared to 29 per cent in the south west of England.

e) **False**   The proportion of smokers in the population is falling. Between 1972 and 1986, it fell from 52 per cent to 35 per cent for males, and from 41 to 31 per cent for females. There is still however a concerning proportion of schoolchildren who smoke and in this group girls are more likely to take up smoking than boys. The habit is most likely to develop between the ages of 14 and 15.

Q45 In acute pericarditis:

a) pain is unaffected by posture

b) pain is often pleuritic in nature

c) is associated with concave upwards ST segment elevation in the anterior chest leads but not in the standard leads of the electrocardiogram

d) anticoagulants are contra-indicated

e) in viral pericarditis, viral culture of pericardial fluid is usually positive

Q46 Concerning acute dissection of the aorta:

a) CT scanning is more likely than echocardiography to be diagnostic

b) urgent surgical correction is more commonly needed in type I than in type III

c) associated aortic valve incompetance commonly develops at some time during this condition

d) characteristically the pain produced radiates anteriorly and up to the left shoulder

e) during repair it is essential to identify the re-entry site of the dissection before surgery can be attempted

A45

a) **False**   One of the characteristics of pericardial pain is that it is profoundly affected by posture. The patient is often most comfortable lying in one particular position.

b) **True**   Pericardial pain is often difficult to differentiate from pleuritic pain and frequently radiates to the shoulders. This is probably produced by irritation of the diaphragm following acute pericardial inflammation.

c) **False**   The characteristic ST segment elevation seen on the electrocardiogram is widespread and is always seen in all leads. If mild ST segment elevation is only seen in the chest leads then this may be more suggestive of a physiological variant rather than true pericarditis.

d) **True**   Anticoagulants are contraindicated in acute pericarditis because of the risk of a haemopericardium.

e) **False**   Several studies have shown that it is impossible to culture viruses from pericardial fluid at any stage of an acute viral pericarditis.

A46

a) **True**   CT scanning has been shown to be the most useful test in this condition both for making the diagnosis and for identifying the re-entry site in the descending aorta. Echocardiography is usually not useful unless there is significant aortic route dilatation and/or associated aortic incompetence.

b) **True**   Proximal dissections (Type I) much more commonly require surgical intervention than distal (Type III) dissections.

c) **True**   Aortic incompetance frequently develops during this condition because of proximal extension of the aortic root tear.

d) **False**   Back pain rather than anterior chest wall or shoulder pain is associated with acute dissection.

e) **False**   Surgical treatment is directed to the area of the proximal tear often in combination with aortic valve replacement. It is not essential to identify the re-entry site. This can be identified and possibly dealt with at a later date.

Q47 During 24 hour Holter monitoring:

a) the subject should not exert himself

b) ventricular tachycardia can be mimicked by the subject "scratching" the electrode

c) slowing of the tape during recording may mimic a bradycardia

d) in patients with hypertrophic cardiomyopathy, asymptomatic ventricular tachycardia can be diagnosed

e) slowing of the tape during playback may mimic A-V conduction abnormalities

Q48 2D echocardiography:

a) can visualise the proximal portions of coronary arteries

b) can detect left ventricular aneurysms

c) can detect ventricular septal defects

d) can effectively exclude bacterial endocarditis

e) cannot detect valve ring abscesses

A47

a) **False** When ambulatory 24 hour Holter monitoring is being performed, the patient should be encouraged to undertake normal daily activities.

b) **True** Artefacts can result from mechanical stimulation of loose electrodes, so it is essential that the electrodes be applied securely by an experienced cardiac technician.

c) **False** Battery failure and slowing of the tape speed as the ECG is being recorded results in an apparent tachycardia rather than a bradycardia.

d) **True** This investigation is an important one in patients with hypertrophic cardiomyopathy, as it has been shown that they suffer arrhythmic deaths. If symptomatic or asymptomatic ventricular tachycardia is discovered, it is essential to start these patients on amiodarone therapy.

e) **True** Slowing of the tape on playback can cause an apparent bradycardia and can suggest conduction abnormalities which are only artefacts.

A48

a) **True** During careful examination of the ascending aorta, the proximal portions of both coronary arteries can be well visualised.

b) **True** This technique is particularly useful in determining global left ventricular function and in diagnosing the presence or absence of left ventricular aneurysms.

c) **True** This technique is useful in the detection of ventricular septal defects and when combined with colour flow measurements, can pick up even very small defects.

d) **False** It should be emphasised that this technique should not be used to exclude bacterial endocarditis. Repeated blood culture is a much more important technique for the diagnosis of this condition.

e) **False** This technique can be useful to detect valvular vegetations, especially when large. Echo-dense areas near valve rings can be diagnostic of valve ring abscesses, which can develop into pseudo-aneurysms.

*Q*49 Cholesterol and coronary artery disease:

a) one in 500 individuals have familial hypercholesterolaemia

b) serum cholesterol increases with age

c) 70 per cent of the UK population have a serum cholesterol of more than 5.2 mmol/l

d) the recommended ratio of daily intake of polyunsaturated to saturated fats (P/S ratio) should be less than 0.3

e) the recommended daily intake of total dietry fat should be 35 per cent of the total energy intake

*Q*50 Epidemiology of coronary artery disease:

a) coronary artery disease in the UK accounts for approximately 15,000 deaths annually

b) middle aged to elderly men in the UK are eight times more likely to die from coronary disease, than those in Japan

c) deaths from coronary disease in the UK have fallen at a comparable rate to that in the USA, New Zealand and Finland

d) "overweight" is usually defined as a body mass index of less than 25

e) "overweight" is an independent risk factor for coronary disease

A49

a) **True**   This is an inherited disorder which causes abnormally high levels of blood cholesterol and thus a high risk of early death from coronary disease.

b) **True**   Although younger women have lower cholesterol concentrations than men, after the age of 50 women have appreciably higher concentrations than men.

c) **True**   In a study of 12,000 British adults the average total cholesterol for men was 5.9 mmol/l and for women 5.8 mmol/l. The risk of infarction is lowest at levels below 4.5 mmol/l.

d) **False**   The recommended P/S ratio is 0.45.

e) **True**   In 1988 the daily UK consumption of fat accounted for 42 per cent of total energy intake and it is recommended that this proportion is now reduced to 35 per cent. Similarly the proportion of saturated fat was 17 per cent of total energy consumption and it is recommended that this figure be reduced to 15 per cent.

A50

a) **False**   The figure is approximately 150,000 deaths annually. Many of these will die out of hospital and often as unwitnessed cardiac arrests.

b) **True**   Furthermore men in the UK are twice as likely to die from coronary disease as those in Italy, and three times more likely than those in France.

c) **False**   The death rate in the UK has fallen over the last 20 years, but at a slower rate than other countries.

d) **False**   "Overweight" is defined as a body mass (weight in kg divided by height in metres) greater than 25.

e) **False**   Overweight is associated with hypertension, decreased physical activity and a raised serum cholesterol, but is not an independent risk factor for coronary disease.

Q51 Technical difficulties during echocardiography can occur in:

a) patients with extreme obesity

b) emphysematous patients

c) patients who have had permanent pacemakers implanted

d) pectus excavatum

e) young children

Q52 Recognised complications of mitral valve prolapse include:

a) exercise-induced ventricular arrhythmias

b) infective endocarditis

c) supraventricular extrasystoles

d) atypical chest pain

e) pericarditis

A51

a) **True**   Ultrasonic examination of the heart is difficult in obese patients, as excessive adipose tissue over and around the heart absorbs sound waves.

b) **True**   Air in alveolar tissue is a good absorber of ultrasonic sound waves and therefore emphysematous patients, who have air in front of the heart, are difficult to echo.

c) **False**   These patients present no special technical difficulties during echocardiography, though it may be difficult to actually visualise the pacemaker wire.

d) **True**   This examination is often difficult in patients with skeletal chest abnormalities.

e) **False**   These patients are particularly easy to echo and high quality tracings are often obtainable as the heart is such a short distance from the ultrasound transducer. There is never obstructive obesity or emphesema. Echocardiography has revolutionised paediatric cardiology and made cardiac catheterisation less necessary in this group of patients.

A52

a) **True**   Mitral valve prolapse is often associated with both supraventricular and ventricular extrasystoles. These extrasystoles may be induced by exercise. They are usually benign.

b) **True**   Infective endocarditis has been reported in mitral valve prolapse making it necessary to advise dental and other antibiotic prophylaxis patients with this condition.

c) **True**   Benign supraventricular extrasystoles and runs of supraventricular tachycardia are common in this condition.

d) **True**   Atypical chest pain and ischaemic sounding chest pain are both reported in this condition and, happily, both usually respond to beta-blocker therapy.

e) **False**   This condition is not associated with pericarditis.

Q53 Concerning the following arrhythmias:

a) Wolfe Parkinson White syndrome (WPW) is characterised by a prolonged PR interval

b) Lown Ganong Levine syndrome is characterised by a widened QRS complex

c) VT is well recognised in cardiomyopathies

d) ambulatory ECG monitoring is helpful in evaluating tachyarrythmias

e) complete bundle branch block may prolong QRS duration

A53

a) **False** WPW syndrome is characterised by a short PR interval, a widened QRS complex due to the presence of a delta wave and a tendency to paroxysmal SVT.

b) **False** LGL syndrome is characterised by a short PR interval, a normal QRS complex and a tendency to paroxysmal tachycardia.

c) **True** The common causes of ventricular tachycardia are myocardial damage from coronary artery disease and cardiomyopathy.

d) **True** Useful information may be provided from an ambulatory recording, if an arrythmia is demonstrated or if a patient experiences symptoms such as palpitations, light-headedness or syncope which correlate with abnormalities in the electrocardiogram.

e) **True** Complete bundle branch block prolongs QRS duration to 0.12 seconds or longer. In incomplete bundle branch block, the QRS duration is 0.10 to 0.11 seconds.

Q54 Transoesophageal echocardiography is superior to transthoracic echocardiography in the following situations:

a) in patients with advanced chronic obstructive airway disease

b) in cases of left atrial thrombus

c) evaluation of prosthetic mitral valve function

d) monitoring patients during operative procedures

e) examination of the thoracic aorta

*A***54**

a) **True**   Patients with advanced COAD and emphysema usually have a very poor transthoracic window through which the examination is unsatisfactory. TOE (Transoesophageal Echocardiography) does not rely on this window.

b) **True**   This is one of the most important applications of TOE. Transthoracic echocardiography does not visualise the left atrial posterior wall or left atrial appendage in as much detail.

c) **True**   By looking at the prosthetic valve from the atrial side rather than the ventricular side, a better assessment of valve function can be made with regard to mitral regurgitation.

d) **True**   Now TOE is being used routinely in some centres to monitor the patient's cardiac function throughout an operation.

e) **True**   Being next to the aorta, TOE is able to show in great detail the aortic morphology. This is particularly useful in evaluating the presence of dissection.

Q55 Thrombolysis in acute myocardial infarction:

a) thrombolytic therapy reduces mortality only if given within six hours of the onset of symptoms

b) because APSAC is derived from recombinant human protein, it can be given if streptokinase has been prescribed in the previous six months

c) a lack of cardiac enzyme rise after treatment suggests that successful reperfusion has occured

d) rtPA can be given if there is history of active peptic ulceration

e) recent stroke is a contraindication to thrombolytic therapy

Q56 Indications for the implantation of a permanent pacemaker include:

a) syncope of undetermined cause

b) congenital symptomatic A-V block

c) carotid sinus hypersensitivity complicated by symptomatic bradycardia

d) symptomatic long pauses in a patient with atrial fibrillation

e) bifasicular block

A55

a) **False**   Evidence from the ISIS2 study showed benefit if thrombolytic therapy is given up to 24 hours after the onset of symptoms. However, the risk/benefit ratio decreases dramatically after 6 hours.

b) **False**   APSAC is equally likely to produce allergic reaction as streptokinase. In these circumstances, rtPA should be given.

c) **False**   An enzyme rise would be expected even after successful reperfusion because of a washout effect.

d) **False**   Any thrombolytic agent is contraindicated.

e) **True**   This applies irrespective of whether the stroke is considered to be haemorrhagic or thrombotic/embolic.

A56

a) **False**   It would be wrong to proceed early to permanent pacemaker implantation in a patient with syncope of underdetermined cause. Other medical conditions such as diabetes and epilepsy should be carefully excluded.

b) **True**   Patients with congential heart block and symptoms related to this heart block will improve following the implantation of a permanent pacemaker. Although permanent implants are not always needed in this group of patients, they have a higher incidence than the general population.

c) **True**   It is now well documented that carotid sinus hypersensitivity resulting in significant bradycardia is considerably improved following the implantation of a permanent pacemaker.

d) **True**   In a patient with symptomatic long pauses in atrial fibrillation with a slow ventricular response on no treatment, permanent pacemaker implantation will produce considerable symptomatic improvement.

e) **False**   In the absence of symptoms bifasicular block is not an indication for a permanent pacemaker implantation.

*Q*57 Primary pulmonary hypertension:

a)   is always of unknown etiology

b)   is usually a congenital condition

c)   is more common amongst women

d)   may deteriorate during pregnancy

e)   may be associated with Raynaud's phenomenon

*Q*58 In primary pulmonary hypertension:

a)   dyspnoea is a common clinical feature

b)   respiratory function tests reveal a Type II defect

c)   lung compliance is well maintained until late

d)   syncope may be the presenting clinical feature

e)   chest pain seldom occurs

*A*57

a) **True**   As it is primary, the etiology of PPH is always unknown. (Do not be confused by ''always'' in this situation.)

b) **False**   PPH with rare exceptions is an acquired condition.

c) **True**   The female-to-male incidence ratio is approximately 3:1.

d) **True**   If this condition is present, it becomes worse during pregnancy.

e) **True**   The common occurrence of Raynaud's phenomenon in association with PPH suggests that both these vascular diseases have a common aetiology.

*A*58

a) **True**   Dyspnoea is the most common symptom of pulmonary hypertension.

b) **False**   Respiratory function tests reveal a Type I defect, i.e. low PO_2 with low or lower normal PCO_2.

c) **False**   Lung compliance is diminished early in the disease process, and there is an early reduction in diffusion capacity.

d) **True**   Syncope can be dramatic in some patients with PPH. Syncope may begin with light-headedness and usually is first noted during or shortly after exercise.

e) **False**   Anginal chest pain is one of the most common features of PPH.

Q59 The following are recognised complications of temporary cardiac pacemaker implantation:

a) post-cardiotomy syndrome

b) asystole

c) the production of an apical pneumothorax

d) myocardial perforation

e) ventricular tachycardia

*A***59**

a) **True**   The insertion of a temporary pacemaker can cause cardiac damage with the production of anti-heart antibodies. The post-cardiotomy syndrome is a recognised complication of the insertion of either a temporary or permanent pacemaker.

b) **True**   In a patient with conducting tissue disease the implantation of a pacemaker can precipitate asystole and require acute resuscitative measures.

c) **True**   This is especially common during "blind" subclavian vein stabs when inserting a temporary wire. The apex of the lung can be perforated, producing a pneumothorax.

d) **True**   Myocardial perforation can occur as a complication of temporary or permanent pacemaker implantation.

e) **True**   Ventricular extrasystoles and runs of ventricular tachycardia can be induced during the temporary pacing procedure, especially when the tricuspid valve is negotiated or when the pacemaker is implanted into the apex of the right ventricle.

*Q*60 Indications for 24 hour ambulatory Holter monitoring include:

a)   syncope and "dizziness"

b)   general fatigue and lethargy

c)   chest pains possibly due to myocardial ischaemia

d)   asymptomatic hypertrophic cardiomyopathy

e)   monitoring the effect and use of anti-arrhythmic drugs

A60

a) True Such symptoms, particularly in elderly patients, may well be due to conducting tissue abnormalities which can often be detected by this investigation. These patients often respond to the implantation of a permanent pacemaker.

b) False There are many causes for these complaints, including psychological problems. Such symptoms are certainly not highly suggestive of conducting tissue abnormalities.

c) True Holter monitoring has now been shown to be as reliable as exercises testing for the detection of symptomatic ischaemic chest pain. It is also useful for the detection of silent myocardial ischaemia. The technique can also be used to assess the efficacy of various anti-anginal preparations.

d) True It is important to look for the occurence of ventricular tachycardia in symptomatic and asymptomatic patients with hypertrophic cardiomyopathy, as they frequently die arrhythmic deaths. These deaths can be prevented by appropriate anti-arrhythmic therapy.

e) True In patients with complicated conducting tissue disease, the efficacy of an anti-arrhythmic drug or various combinations can be assessed by 24 hour continuous ambulatory cardiac monitoring.

Q61 Physical signs suggesting PPH include:

a) left ventricular hypertrophy

b) pulmonary incompetence

c) systolic clicks

d) left-sided fourth heart sound

e) enlarged liver

Q62 Regarding PPH:

a) a routine haematological screen may reveal polycythaemia

b) the pulmonary artery is enlarged

c) 'P' waves may have a characteristic appearance

d) 'T' waves are usually hyperacute

e) cardiac catheterisation is a useful diagnostic tool

A61

a) **False**   Right rather than left ventricular hypertrophy is seen. Left ventricular hypertrophy occurs in systemic hypertension and not in pulmonary hypertension.

b) **True**   Aneurysmal dilation of the main pulmonary artery may lead to pulmonary valve incompetence producing a diastolic murmur along the left sternal border.

c) **True**   Systolic clicks and/or an ejection systolic murmur associated with pulmonary artery dilatation may be audible.

d) **False**   As the right heart is under strain, one would therefore expect to find a right-sided rather than a left-sided fourth heart sound.

e) **True**   Functional tricuspid regurgitation occurs as a result of persistent right ventricular strain. In its severest form, tricuspid regurgitation may produce expansile pulsation of the enlarged liver due to congestion.

A62

a) **True**   Although the routine haematological and chemical examinations are usually normal, occasionally patients have polycythaemia which usually tends to be associated with mild arterial hypoxaemia.

b) **True**   The most prominent feature of the chest radiograph is the enlargement of the main pulmonary artery segment in the PA view. The distal radicles of the pulmonary vascular markings typically are diminished, giving vascular shadows a ''pruned'' appearance.

c) **True**   The 'P' wave is usually abnormally tall (more than 2.5 mm) especially in Lead II and also in Leads III and AVF.

d) **False**   The 'T' waves are inverted and not hyperacute in precordial Leads V1, V2 and V3. Hyperacute 'T' waves are a sign of hyperkalaemia.

e) **True**   Cardiac catheterisation is considered the definitive diagnostic procedure for PPH because it quantifies vascular obstruction and effectively excludes congenital cardiac shunts, defects and mitral valve disease as causes.

Q63 In asymptomatic children the following changes on ambulatory 24 hour Holter monitoring are significant:

a) episodes of second degree A-block with Wenckebach phenomenon

b) episodes of first degree A-V block

c) episodes of atrial tachycardia

d) short non-sustained runs of ventricular tachycardia

e) isolated ventricular extrasystoles

Q64 Serious conducting tissue disease requiring the implantation of a permanent pacemaker:

a) is commonly a result of viral illness

b) can occur following an attack of rheumatic fever

c) can occur as a result of ischaemic heart disease

d) may follow successful cardiac surgery

e) often does not show up on a resting electrocardiogram

A63

a) **False** Such episodes have been well documented to occur in completely normal children and adults.

b) **False** Especially in the absence of symptoms, short episodes of first degree AV block occur in the normal population.

c) **False** Short runs of "benign" atrial tachycardia frequently occur in normal subjects without underlying heart disease.

d) **False** Short runs of ventricular tachycardia can be detected in otherwise healthy individuals with normal hearts.

e) **False** Isolated ventricular extrasystoles occur in up to 75 per cent of healthy subjects.

A64

a) **False** Viruses do attack the heart but more commonly produce ventricular extrasystoles and runs of ventricular tachycardia rather than brady-arrhythmias.

b) **False** Although conducting tissue abnormalities are well documented following an attack of rheumatic fever, this rarely if ever necessitates pacemaker implantation.

c) **True** Ischaemic heart disease may result in tachy-arrhythmias and brady-arrhythmias. If serious conduting tissue disease results then this may require treatment with a combination of pacing and anti-arrhythmic therapy.

d) **True** Following repair of a ventricular septal defect, especially a high membranous VSD, damage to the AV node may be produced resulting in complete block, necessitating the implantation of a permanent pacemaker.

e) **False** Although serious conducting tissue disease can occur in the presence of a normal resting ECG, this is unusual. Much more commonly, evidence of varying degrees of heart block will be seen on the resting electrocardiogram.

Q65 In pulmonary embolism:

a) a majority of the thrombi originate in the lower extremity

b) is the most common cause of an acute respiratory admission to hospital

c) the venous volume of a thrombus in the pelvis is more than in the leg

d) thrombophlebitis does not lead to a pulmonary embolism

e) atrial fibrillation is the most common complicating arrythmia

Q66 The following factors predispose to venous thrombosis:

a) cardiac failure

b) a sedentary occupation

c) typhoid fever

d) SLE

e) pregnancy

A65

a) **True**   In over 90 per cent of cases, venous thromboses that eventually find their way to the lung, form in the calves.

b) **True**   Acute pulmonary embolism is the most common acute pulmonary disease in the adult hospital population.

c) **False**   A clot extending from the calf to the iliac vein has a volume of approximately 100 ml. Another site of clot origin is the pelvis, but its venous volume is much less than that of the legs.

d) **False**   Phlebothrombosis, which is a thrombosis without inflammatory reaction, and thrombophlebitis, a thrombus with inflammatory non-bacterial reaction, both predispose to pulmonary embolism.

e) **True**   The usual electrocardiographic changes found during an acute pulmonary embolus are right axis deviation and right ventricular hypertrophy. The most common arrythmia produced is atrial fibrillation.

A66

a) **True**   Cardiac failure is by far the most important condition predisposing to thromboembolism.

b) **False**   A sedentary occupation alone is rarely a cause of venous thrombosis, but if added to another factor, such as congestive cardiac failure, or smoking, it becomes a highly significant factor.

c) **True**   Typhoid fever is a well-documented cause of thrombosis.

d) **True**   In SLE the production of lupus anticoagulant paradoxically predisposes to clot formation and hence thromboembolism.

e) **True**   A hypercoaguable state occurs during pregnancy, and also when taking the oral contraceptive pill, thus predisposing to thrombus formation.

Q67 In sick sinus syndrome:

a) ventricular pacing is preferable to atrial pacing

b) the use of beta blocking drugs is contraindicated

c) impaired A-V conduction may occur

d) there is an association with systemic emboli

e) similar problems have been reported following diptheria infections

Q68 Contraindications to exercise stress testing include:

a) essential hypertension

b) aortic stenosis

c) pyrexial illness

d) unstable angina

e) acute myocarditis

A67

a) **False**   Atrial pacing rather than ventricular pacing is preferable, especially in young people. It achieves a better cardiac output because the atrial contribution to stroke volume is retained. Atrial pacing is only possible when AV node conduction is normal.

b) **False**   No anti-arrhythmic drugs are contraindicated in this condition, which may require treatment with a combination of permanent pacing and anti-arrhythmic drugs.

c) **True**   Impairment of A-V node conduction is well documented.

d) **True**   An increased incidence of systemic emboli has been shown to occur in patients with the sick sinus syndrome.

e) **True**   Conducting tissue abnormalities are common in patients with acute diptheria infections.

A68

a) **True**   Most exercise testing laboratories do not perform exercise tests on patients with uncontrolled hypertension as exercise is known to elevate the blood pressure and this may result in a CVA.

b) **True**   Aortic stenosis is a definite contraindication to exercise stress testing, which may result in cardiovascular collapse.

c) **True**   Any severe systemic illness with or without a significant pyrexia is a contraindication to exercise stress testing.

d) **True**   Cardiac catheterisation is a preferable investigation in a patient with unstable or crescendo angina.

e) **True**   It is now well proven that patients with myocarditis can experience episodes of ventricular tachycardia during exercise, which should be definitely avoided during the acute infective illness.

*Q*69 Regarding pulmonary embolism:

a)   the distribution of emboli in the lungs is erratic

b)   pulmonary arterial pressure rises as a result of emboli

c)   revascularisation may occur within minutes

d)   pulmonary embolism may occur during sudden exertion

e)   usually produces a characteristic pattern on the ECG

*Q*70 Pulmonary embolism:

a)   is found in approximately 5 per cent of routine post mortems

b)   increases in its incidence with age

c)   affects women to men in a ratio of 2:1

d)   approximately 50 per cent die within 1 hour

e)   hypercapnoea is common

*A*69

a) **False**   The distribution of emboli in the lungs follows closely the distribution of blood flow, i.e. mainly in the lower lobes of the lungs.

b) **True**   The obstruction to the normal flow of blood to the lungs causes a rise in pulmonary aterial pressure.

c) **True**   As the pressure in the pulmonary artery rises, blood forces its way through the clot so that partial revascularisation occurs within minutes.

d) **True**   Although the immediate cause of emboli formation is usually not apparent, it sometimes occurs on arising from bed, straining at stool, exertion or hyperventilation. All of these activities can result in distension of the leg veins, thereby promoting clot displacement.

e) **False**   The $S_1Q_3T_3$ pattern only occurs in about 10 per cent of patients with an acute pulmonary embolus. The most common ECG abnormality is atrial fibrillation.

*A*70

a) **False**   Pulmonary emboli are an extremely common finding at post mortem. They are found in approximately 10 per cent of all post mortems in general hospitals, and 25 per cent in hospitals giving palliative care.

b) **True**   The incidence of pulmonary embolism increases with age, being rare under 20 and infrequent under 30. It becomes progressively more common with advancing age.

c) **False**   There is an equal sex incidence.

d) **False**   Approximately 10 per cent of patients with PE die almost immediately or within the first hour.

e) **False**   In pulmonary embolism there is a Type I respiratory failure, i.e. low PO_2 with low or normal PCO_2.

Q71 The following can produce false positive results on exercise stress testing:

a) beta-blockers

b) digoxin

c) hypertension with LV hypertrophy

d) anaemia

e) calcium antagonists

Q72 The following changes can be taken as normal physiological variants during exercise testing:

a) right axis deviation

b) the development of left bundle-branch block

c) multifocal ventricular extrasystoles

d) enlargement of the P Wave in Standard Leads II and III

e) shortening of the P R interval

*A*71

a) **False**   Beta-blockers may abolish resting T Wave abnormalities and can increase the specificity of exercise stress testing by reducing the incidence of false positive results.

b) **True**   Digoxin is well known to cause false positive results through its affect on ST segment changes.

c) **True**   Hypertension with re-polarisation changes resulting in ST segment depression can produce false positive stress tests.

d) **True**   Anaemia will cause false positive results in patients with normal coronary arteries although myocardial ischaemia does not occur as a result of the anaemia.

e) **False**   Calcium antagonist drugs do not have any effects on repolarisation changes. They are quite safe to continue during exercise testing in patients who are suspected of having angina pectoris.

*A*72

a) **True**   Right axis deviation can occur during exercise testing and this is a normal physiological variation. The development of right bundle branch block, however, is usually abnormal.

b) **False**   The development of left bundle branch block signifies probable myocardial ischaemia.

c) **False**   The development of ventricular extrasystoles during exercise, especially if these have multifocal origins, is thought to signify ischaemic heart disease. Ventricular extrasystoles which occur at rest (and are abolished by exercise), particularly if they are unifocal, are considered benign.

d) **True**   During exercise, right axis deviation of the P Wave occurs so that it becomes taller in Standard Leads II and III.

e) **True**   This is a normal physiological variation related to tachycardia produced by exercise.

Q73 Late complications of insertion of a permanent pacemaker include:

a) skin ulceration over the implant site

b) development of localised myocarditis

c) infective endocarditis

d) wire fracture

e) post-cardiotomy syndrome

*A*73

a) **True**   Skin ulceration over the permanent pacemaker generator is not uncommon and seems to be related to chronic rejection of the metal used to cover the pacemaker box rather than long-term infection. It usually necessitates re-implantation of the pacemaker on the other side of the chest and eventually may require implantation of an epicardial system.

b) **False**   Myocarditis has never been reported following permanent pacemaker implantation.

c) **True**   Infective endocarditis is a rare recognised complication following the insertion of a permanent pacemaker.

d) **True**   Constant handling of the generator – "Twiddler's Syndrome" – can lead to fracture of the wire especially if it is possible to rotate the generator in its pocket.

e) **True**   Cardiac damage produced by electrode implantation may result in the generation of anti-heart antibodies and pericardiac pain due to the post-cardiotomy syndrome.

Q74

Are the following significant findings, on routine examination of a fit thirty year old man:

a)   extrasystoles

b)   early, short systolic bruit at left sternal edge

c)   early, short diastolic bruit at left sternal edge

d)   bundle-branch block

e)   split heart sound at mitral area

A74

a) **False**   In the absence of myocardial or valvular heart disease extrasystoles are a common finding in the normal heart.

b) **False**   An early, short systolic bruit at the left sternal edge is usually benign and normal. The main pathological problem to be excluded is aortic valve stenosis: this should be done by careful palpation of the pulse, listening for the presence of the aortic component of the second heart sound and establishing the absence of an aortic valve click and an early diastolic murmur suggestive of concomitant aortic valve incompetence.

c) **True**   An early, short diastolic bruit, on the other hand, is pathological and suggestive of either pulmonary valve incompetence or, more frequently, aortic valve incompetence in association with an abnormal and probably bicuspid aortic valve.

d) **True**   The question on bundle-branch block is difficult, as sometimes **right** bundle-branch block can be physiological and benign. However, in the vast majority of cases it is pathological, the most common cause being cor polmonale associated with cigarette smoking. **Left** bundle-branch block is most commonly associated with specific cardiac disease, either ischaemic or valvular. In the absence of further information, this question should be marked as being significant of possible pathology, warranting further investigations.

e) **True**   The last question is a "trick question" relating to a well-known cardiological faux pas. Split second heart sounds are never heard in the mitral area. If there appears to be such a sound, it is more likely to be an additional diastolic sound, most commonly due to an opening snap. This is therefore a very significant finding in a fit young man and warrants further investigations and certainly an echocardiogram.

Q75 Pulsus alternans:

a)   is best recognised on the electrocardiogram

b)   indicates bad prognosis

c)   is associated with diastolic gallop

d)   is seen with restrictive pericarditis

e)   causes an additional sound in diastole

Q76 In Wolfe-Parkinson-White syndrome:

a)   there is often a history of rheumatic fever

b)   the PR interval is prolonged

c)   the QRS time is prolonged

d)   there is usually tall T Waves

e)   there is generally an increased tendency toward paroxysmal tachycardia

*A*75

a) **False**   Pulsus alternans is a sign of a severely abnormal left ventricle. It indicates gross left ventricular failure and almost always is associated with early demise of the patient. It is certainly not best recognised on the ECG.

b) **True**   It certainly does always indicate a bad prognosis.

c) **True**   Because of the left ventricular failure, there is always an associated diastolic gallop.

d) **False**   The pulse abnormality associated with this condition is pulsus paradoxus, which is a very different physical sign.

e) **True**   There is invariably an additional sound in diastole, either a third or fourth heart sound or, more commonly, a summation gallop if the patient is still in sinus rhythm.

*A*76

a) **False**   The W-P-W syndrome is a congenitally inherited aberrant conducting pathway, which is absolutely nothing to do with rheumatic fever.

b) **False**   It is a high speed conducting tissue pathway that by definition always produces a short PR interval.

c) **True**   The QRS time is always prolonged because of the slanting upwards so called "delta wave" that is often seen in this condition.

d) **False**   Tall T waves may occur in this condition, but they are certainly not a common find. Indeed, anything can happen to the ST segment or the T wave in this condition because, basically, anything that produces abnormal depolarisation, will produce abnormal repolarisation changes which are manifest in the ST segment and/or T wave. Certainly, tall T waves are not a particularly recognised feature of this syndrome.

e) **True**   An increased liability to paroxysmal tachycardia is the main problem in this condition and it may well be essentially asymptomatic or, on the other hand, may produce symptoms of palpitation, dizziness and syncopy. In extreme conditions it may result in sudden death.

Q77 When treating rheumatic heart disease:

a) symptomatic mitral stenosis may be treated medically for many years

b) aortic valvuloplasty is the treatment of choice in aortic stenosis

c) a gradient of 85 mmHg in aortic stenosis in indicative of mild to moderate disease

d) uncontrolled infective endocarditis is an indication for surgery in mitral stenosis.

e) haemolysis may be a complication of prosthetic valve replacement

Q78 In mixed mitral valve disease stenosis is likely to be "dominant" when:

a) there is a loud first heart sound

b) the apex beat is located in the anterior axillary line

c) a third heart sound is heard

d) the pulse is irregularly irregular

e) the apex beat has a tapping quality

A77

a) **True**   Symptoms can be controlled with the use of diuretics, ACE inhibitors and anticoagulants where appropriate.

b) **False**   Valvuloplasty is sometimes used but often with poor results and aortic valve replacement is the treatment of choice in most cases.

c) **False**   A gradient of 85 mmHg indicates moderate to severe disease.

d) **True**   This is an absolute indication for valve replacement.

e) **True**   Sometimes haemolysis can occur as a result of trauma to the red blood cells when pressing through the prosthetic valve.

A78

a) **True**   A loud first heart sound is consistent with stenosis.

b) **False**   An enlarged heart suggests significant regurgitation.

c) **False**   A third heart sound is not present in severe stenosis as the atrial impulse is not sufficiently transmitted to the ventricle.

d) **False**   Atrial fibrillation is a common arrhythmia in both mitral stenosis and regurgitation and is not particularly associated with one rather than the other.

e) **True**   This is caused by a loud first heart sound.

Q79 The chest X-ray in rheumatic heart disease may reveal:

a) cardiomegaly more commonly in mitral stenosis than in mitral regurgitation

b) cardiomegaly in aortic regurgitation

c) elevation of the left main bronchus in mitral stenosis

d) oligaemic lung fields in pulmonary stenosis

e) a double right heart border in mitral regurgitation

Q80 Pulmonary hypertension:

a) causes the pulmonary and aortic components of the second heart sound to be further apart

b) is a cause of a Graham-Steel murmur

c) can cause peripheral cyanosis

d) is a cause of atrial fibrillation

e) gives rise to giant A waves in the JVP

*A***79**   *a)* **False**   Mitral regurgitation more frequently causes cardiomegaly; the left atrium may enlarge in mitral stenosis.

b) **True**   Longstanding aortic regurgitation will cause left ventricular enlargement.

c) **True**   Left atrial enlargement in mitral stenosis can cause widening of the carina and elevation of the left main bronchus.

d) **True**   Reduced blood flow will cause oligaemic lung fields.

e) **True**   Longstanding mitral regurgitation can produce left atrial enlargement, one sign of which is a double right heart shadow.

*A***80**   *a)* **False**   The pulmonary component becomes closer to the aortic component of the second heart sound as the pulmonary hypertension becomes more severe.

b) **True**   The pulmonary valve becomes incompetent causing a Graham-Steel murmur.

c) **True**   This is due to the low cardiac output.

d) **True**   This is usually a relatively late complication.

e) **True**   Right atrial systole has to overcome an increased right ventricular end diastolic pressure.

Q81 Aortic regurgitation:

a) can cause left ventricular hypertrophy detectable on the ECG

b) when severe can partially close the anterior mitral valve leaflet

c) is sometimes caused by a ventricular septal defect

d) is a cause of giant V waves in the JVP

e) is often associated with Kussmaul's sign

Q82 In acute rheumatic fever:

a) Aschoff's bodies are pathognomic

b) the vegetations on valve leaflets are large, friable and often give rise to embolic manifestations

c) a Carey-Coombs murmur may be heard

d) the PR interval is prolonged

e) the aortic valve is most frequently involved

*A*81

a) **True**   Longstanding aortic regurgitation gives rise to left ventricular hypertrophy.

b) **True**   It is this which produces the Austin Flint murmur.

c) **True**   Occasionally, particularly in high membranous ventricular septal defects, the aortic valve is not sufficiently supported and one or more of its cusps are liable to prolapse.

d) **False**   Tricuspid regurgitation produces giant V waves in the JVP.

e) **False**   Kussmaul's sign is found in pericardial tamponade.

*A*82

a) **True**   These consist of a central necrotic area surrounded by epitheliod cells and lymphocytes.

b) **False**   The vegetations tend to be small and firmly attached and therefore rarely embolize.

c) **True**   This is an apical diastolic murmur caused by thickened mitral valve leaflets.

d) **True**   The PR interval is often prolonged; however, heart block is not usually a clinical problem.

e) **False**   The aortic valve is the second most frequently affected, the mitral valve being the first.

Q83 In pericardial tamponade:

a)   a frictional rub is heard in the majority of cases

b)   the central venous pressure increases on inspiration

c)   the apex beat is usually heaving in character

d)   the systemic blood pressure falls on inspiration

e)   fine basal crepitations are often heard at the lung bases

Q84 Aortic stenosis:

a)   is likely to be subvalvular when a click is audible

b)   caused a low blood pressure and narrow pulse pressure

c)   is a cause of giant A waves in the JVP

d)   causes paradoxical splitting of S_2

e)   often causes a left parasternal heave

A83

a) **False**   A friction rub is not heard as the pericardial layers are separated by the effusion.

b) **True**   During deep inspiration there is an increased venous return to the right side of the heart. When pericardial tamponade is present the right ventricle is unable to accommodate this increased volume, therefore the JVP rises with deep inspiration. This is known as Kussmaul's sign.

c) **False**   The apex beat may not be palpable in many cases.

d) **True**   This is pulsus paradoxus.

e) **True**   The resulting low cardiac output causes pulmonary oedema.

A84

a) **False**   An ejection click indicates a valvular origin.

b) **True**   Both these clinical signs are frequently present in moderate to severe cases of aortic stenosis.

c) **False**   Tricuspid stenosis and right ventricular outflow obstruction are causes of giant A waves.

d) **True**   Obstruction of left ventricular outflow causes delayed aortic valve closure.

e) **False**   A left parasternal heave results from right ventricular hypertrophy,

Q85 When assessing the arterial pulse:

a) pulses alternans is associated with constrictive pericarditis

b) a slow rising, plateau pulse is usually found in hypertrophic obstructive cardiomyopathy

c) a collapsing pulse is diagnostic of aortic incompetence

d) a bisferens pulse is found in severe mixed aortic valve disease

e) Corrigan's pulse is best felt in the left brachial artery

Q86 On assessing the heart sounds:

a) a split S_1 can often be physiological

b) reversed splitting of S_2 is characteristic of an ostium secundum defect

c) the second heart sound is loud in coarctation of the aorta

d) wide reversed splitting of S_2 occurs in right bundle branch block

e) a loud S_3 is heard in constrictive pericarditis

*A*85

a) **False** Pulsus alternans is associated with left ventricular failure.

b) **False** Hypertrophic obstructive cardiomyopathy gives rise to a jerky pulse.

c) **False** A collapsing pulse can be caused by a large patent ductus arteriosus.

d) **True** This is most marked in moderate stenosis and severe regurgitation.

e) **False** A Corrigan's pulse is the bounding pulse seen in the neck.

*A*86

a) **True** In 85 per cent of healthy people the first heart sound is split.

b) **False** Fixed splitting of the second heart sound is a pathopneumonic physical sign, found in both ostium primum and secundum atrial septal defects.

c) **True** The second heart sound is loud in coarctation of the aorta because of the proximal hypertension.

d) **False** There is a wide splitting of the second heart sound in right bundle branch block.

e) **True** This is sometimes known as a pericardial knock.

Q87 An apical mid-diastolic murmur:

a)   is produced by a left atrial myxoma

b)   can be a Carey-Coombs murmur

c)   can be associated with severe aortic regurgitation

d)   in severe mitral stenosis is associated with a loud S_3

e)   is accentuated after exercise

Q88 Mitral regurgitation:

a)   produces an apical ejection systolic murmur radiating to the axilla

b)   can produce a systolic apical thrill

c)   is a cause of giant V waves in the JVP

d)   can cause a double shadow on the right heart border

e)   is typically associated with a pulsatile liver

A87

a) **True** — A left atrial myxoma frequently produces intermittent obstruction of the mitral valve in diastole. It is most commonly associated with a mid to late apical diastolic murmur.

b) **True** — The so called Carey-Coombs murmur is a mid diastolic murmur produced by mitral valvulitis in an attack of acute rheumatic fever.

c) **True** — This Austin Flint murmur is caused by the regurgitant jet partially closing the anterior mitral valve leaflet.

d) **False** — A third heart sound is not produced by mitral stenosis. It is present in moderate to severe mitral regurgitation, when it is frequently very loud.

e) **True** — This is because the flow across the valve in mitral stenosis is increased.

A88

a) **False** — The murmur is pansystolic in nature.

b) **True** — This is present when the regurgitation is severe.

c) **False** — Tricuspid regurgitation causes giant V waves.

d) **True** — Longstanding mitral regurgitation results in enlargement of the left atrium, which can cause a double right heart border seen on a PA chest X-ray.

e) **False** — Tricuspid regurgitation results in a pulsatile liver.

Q89 An early diastolic murmur:

a)   may be associated with Duroziez's Sign

b)   may be a normal finding in a fit young man

c)   is often accompanied by bifid P waves on the ECG

d)   is a common, usually insignificant, finding in a person with chest pain

e)   is a well recognised finding in patients with seronegative arthritis

Q90 In mitral stenosis:

a)   there is characteristically a loud S_2 and an opening snap

b)   the closer the opening snap is to M_1 the more severe is the stenosis

c)   presystolic accentuation of the diastolic murmur can occur in the presence of atrial fibrillation

d)   a right sided hemiparesis can be the presenting sign

e)   pulmonary haemosiderosis can ocur, particularly in the mid and lower zone

A89

a) **True** This is when a diastolic murmur is heard over the femoral artery which is partially obstructed with a finger distal to the stethoscope.

b) **False** Early diastolic murmurs are always pathological and indicate either aortic or pulmonary valvular regurgitation.

c) **False** Bifid P waves are caused by left atrial hypertrophy which is often associated with mitral valve disease.

d) **False** This murmur may indicate aortic incompetence secondary to a dissecting aortic aneurysm.

e) **True** Aortic regurgitation is associated with ankylosing spondylitis and other similar diseases.

A90

a) **False** There is often an audible opening snap but it is S_1 which is characteristically loud. It can be quiet, however, if the valve is immobile.

b) **False** The closer the opening snap is to the second the more severe is the stenosis.

c) **True** Presystolic accentuation is thought to be caused by increasing turbulance of blood flow as the valve leaflets come together.

d) **True** Systemic emolization is frequent, particularly when the left atrium is enlarged and atrial fibrillation is present.

e) **True** This is seen after repeated episodes of interstitial pulmonary oedema.

Q91 In tricuspid regurgitation:

a) there is a wide systemic pulse pressure

b) the murmur is best heard on inspiration

c) a giant A wave is produced in the venous pulse

d) ascites may be produced

e) bacterial endocarditis may be a cause

Q92 An ejection systolic murmur:

a) is heard in aortic stenosis

b) is a common finding in a young person with pyrexial illness

c) is present at the lower left sternal edge in tricuspid regurgitation

d) is heard in the presence of an atrial septal defect

e) is caused by ventricular septal defects

*A*91

a) **False**   There is a wide pulse pressure in aortic incompetence.

b) **True**   Murmurs on the right side of the heart are best heard on inspiration.

c) **False**   A giant V wave is produced in the jugular venous pulse.

d) **True**   Also the liver is enlarged and pulsatile.

e) **True**   Particularly when it is secondary to septicaemia from intravenous drug abuse.

*A*92

a) **True**   It is heard maximally in the aortic area and left sternal edge.

b) **True**   An aortic ejection murmur without any other features of aortic stenosis is a common benign feature in anybody with a severe pyrexial illness.

c) **False**   Tricuspid regurgitation produces a pan systolic murmur.

d) **True**   Is produced by the increased flow across the pulmonary valve.

e) **False**   Ventricular septal defects cause pansystolic murmurs.

Q93 On palpation of the precordium:

a) the apex beat is usually laterally displaced in severe mitral stenosis

b) the second heart sound is usually palpable as a tapping apex beat in mitral stenosis

c) there is sometimes a double apical impulse with a left ventricular aneurysm

d) the apex beat can be laterally displaced in the presence of an early diastolic murmur

e) a left parasternal heave can be associated with a palable pulmonary component of the second heart sound

Q94 The A wave of the JVP:

a) occurs immediately after S_1

b) is absent in atrial fibrillation

c) is particularly large in tricuspid regurgitation

d) is large in pulmonary artery hypertension

e) is caused by right atrial filling

*A*93

a) **False**   The apex beat is not usually palpable in even severe mitral stenosis because the left ventricle is quite small in this condition. On the other hand the apex beat is frequently laterally displaced in moderate to severe mitral regurgitation.

b) **False**   The first heart sound is often palpable as a tapping apex beat is mitral stenosis.

c) **True**   The impulse from the aneurysm can be asynchronous with the apex beat.

d) **True**   The left ventricle dilates with significant aortic incompetence.

e) **True**   In pulmonary hypertension usually with associated right ventricular hypertrophy, there may frequently be a palpable pulmonary component to the S_2.

*A*94

a) **False**   The A wave occurs immediately prior to S_1 as it is due to right atrial contraction, which is prior to cessation of flow across the mitral and tricuspid valves.

b) **True**   There is no organised atrial contraction in AF and therefore no A wave is produced.

c) **False**   There is a large V wave in tricuspid regurgitation.

d) **True**   The A wave is enlarged when right atrial outflow is obstructed.

e) **False**   The A wave is caused by right atrial contraction.

Q95 On examining a hypertensive patient:

a) atrial flutter may be associated with hypertensive heart disease

b) retinal microaneurysms indicate grade three hypertensive retinopathy

c) renal bruits are often present

d) moon shaped facies may be relevant

e) very large hands may be aetiologically important

Q96 Acute rheumatic fever:

a) is generally a very rare disease

b) over the last 10 years has been produced or associated with penicillin resistant streptococci

c) may cause erythema marginatum which may remain pruritic for several days

d) may cause nodules which appear over tendons and bony prominences

e) may present as Sydenham's Chorea which can have a latent period of up to six months after the streptococcal infection

*A*95

a) **True**   Atrial flutter can be a part of hypertensive heart disease.

b) **False**   Grade three hypertensive retinopathy consists of flame shaped haemorrhages and microinfarcts. Microaneurysms are found in diabetic retinopathy.

c) **False**   Renal bruits indicative of renal artery stenosis are only rarely discovered in hypertensive patients.

d) **True**   moon shaped facies may suggest a diagnosis of Cushings Syndrome.

e) **True**   Acromegaly causes hands to be enlarged and is a cause of hypertension.

*A*96

a) **False**   Acute rheumatic fever is still a problem on a world scale.

b) **False**   To date the Lancefield Group A, Griffiths Type 12 strep viridans, associated with acute rheumatic fever, has not been found resistant to penicillin.

c) **False**   Erythema marginatum is usually only present for twenty-four hours although it may recur. It is not pruritic.

d) **True**   Rheumatic nodules do occur in this distribution.

e) **True**   Sydenham's Chorea may occur from one to six months after infection and may or may not be associated with carditis or arthritis.

Q97 In Fallot's tetralogy:

a) clubbing is rare

b) growth is retarded

c) syncope is a common symptom

d) a pansystolic murmur is usual

e) P2 is loud

Q98 Concerning infective endocarditis:

a) streptococcus viridans is now a rare cause of this condition

b) it can occur following an attack of "Q fever"

c) it may occur on a normal aortic valve

d) it is now most commonly a disease of the over-sixties

e) clubbing is found in about 60 per cent of cases

A97

a) **False**   Clubbing is common.

b) **True**   This is due to peripheral oxygen tissue desaturation.

c) **True**   This may occur due to low cardiac output and/or tachyarrythmias.

d) **False**   The classical murmur heard in this condition is an ejection systolic pulmonary murmur, due to pulmonary valve and infundibular stenosis.

e) **False**   P2 is soft, inaudible or even absent in some cases.

A98

a) **False**   Strepococcus viridans (non-haemolytic) is still the commonest cause of this condition in the UK (45 per cent). The most usual source is the teeth.

b) **True**   Coxiella Burnetii (''Q fever'') is a well-documented but rare cause of infective endocarditis.

c) **True**   Healthy valves are infected during a severe septicaemia and may account for up to 50 per cent of cases.

d) **True**   This disease used to be most common in young adults (aged 20 to 30) with rheumatic or congenital heart disease, but it is now more commonly found in the over-sixties.

e) **False**   Clubbing of the fingers occurs in about 20 per cent of cases.

Q99 Acute pericarditis:

a) may be the first indication of SLE

b) constrictive pericarditis is not uncommon following a severe attack of rheumatic fever

c) is common in acute renal failure

d) often produces an abnormal chest X-ray

e) is best diagnosed by echocardiography

Q100 Concerning syphilitic aortitis:

a) angina is a common symptom

b) coughing may occur

c) an absent left radial pulse is a common complication

d) is a frequent complication of congenital syphilis

e) responds well to intramuscular penicillin injections

A 99

a) **True**   Pericarditis is a common complication of SLE. It may occur early in severe cases.

b) **False**   Rheumatic fever produces a severe pericarditis, but this is always serous rather than fibrinous. It therefore never organises nor calcifies to produce constriction.

c) **True**   A pericardial rub is a common finding in uraemic patients.

d) **False**   The chest X-ray is usually normal in acute pericarditis.

e) **False**   Echocardiography is unhelpful in acute pericarditis as the small quantity of pericardial fluid present is usually undetectable.

A 100

a) **True**   Fifty per cent of patients are affected with angina, which is often severe.

b) **True**   Coughing is a common complication, usually due to aneurysmal dilatation of the arch of the aorta, with compression of the trachea and of the recurrent laryngeal nerve.

c) **True**   As above. The aneurysmal aorta may compress and block the left subclavian artery.

d) **False**   Congenital syphilis never produces aortitis.

e) **False**   At this stage penicillin will not be of any use and may indeed be harmful, possibly causing anaphylaxis.